Migraine Mastery: Understanding, Managing, and Overcoming the Pain

-B.R.THATAVARTHI

Published by Amazon KDP

<u>**Disclaimer:**</u>

The information provided in this book, "Migraine Mastery: Understanding, Managing, and Overcoming the Pain," is intended solely for informational purposes. The content presented in this book is not a substitute for professional medical advice, diagnosis, or treatment. It is important to consult with qualified healthcare professionals before making any decisions related to your health, especially if you are dealing with migraine or any other medical condition.

The author and publisher of this book have made reasonable efforts to ensure the accuracy and completeness of the information presented. However, they do not guarantee the accuracy or applicability of the content to individual cases. Every person's health situation is unique, and what might be suitable for one individual may not be appropriate for another.

Readers are encouraged to use their discretion and judgment when applying the information from this book to their own circumstances. The author and publisher shall not be held liable for any damages or consequences arising from the use of this book's information. It is strongly recommended to seek professional medical guidance before implementing any changes to your healthcare routine based on the content of this book.

By reading this book, you acknowledge and agree to the above disclaimer.

Content

1.Introduction to Migraines

In the realm of human experiences, few phenomena can match the perplexing nature of migraines. Migraines are not merely headaches; they are intricate neurological events that weave a complex tapestry of sensations, symptoms, and challenges for those who endure them. Like silent storms within the brain, migraines can disrupt lives, alter plans, and cast a shadow over even the brightest moments. This book delves into the fascinating world of migraines, aiming to demystify their enigmatic nature and provide insights into understanding, managing, and navigating the intricate paths of this condition.

Migraines are far from being a modern ailment; they have been a part of human history for centuries. From the ancient civilizations that grappled with their presence to the contemporary scientific breakthroughs that shed light on their underlying mechanisms, migraines have persisted as both a medical puzzle and a deeply personal experience. The pages that follow seek to embrace the dual perspective of medical exploration and individual stories, combining the empirical with the emotional to offer a comprehensive understanding of migraines.

In this journey, we will embark upon a multidimensional exploration. We will uncover the physiological intricacies that trigger migraines, exploring the intertwining factors of genetics, environment, and brain chemistry. We will delve into the kaleidoscope of symptoms that accompany these episodes—throbbing pain, visual disturbances, nausea, and sensitivity to light and sound, among others—painting a vivid picture of the myriad ways migraines can manifest. But we will also acknowledge the subtleties that often go unnoticed, the hidden struggles that only those who experience migraines firsthand truly comprehend.

Yet, this book is not solely about the challenges. It is also about empowerment and resilience. Armed with the latest medical insights and practical advice, individuals with migraines can navigate their lives with greater agency. By understanding triggers, adopting healthy lifestyle choices, and harnessing the power of treatments, sufferers can regain a sense of control over their experiences. Moreover, loved ones, friends, and colleagues can develop empathy and comprehension, fostering a more supportive environment for those facing migraines.

As we progress through these chapters, it's important to remember that migraines are not monolithic; they are as diverse as the individuals who experience them. Each story shared, each medical discovery unveiled, contributes to a richer tapestry of knowledge. Together, we can embrace the complexity of migraines, emboldened by the desire to comprehend, empathize, and ultimately transform the narrative surrounding this condition.

So, whether you are someone who grapples with migraines, a caregiver seeking understanding, a medical professional striving to provide comprehensive care, or simply a curious soul looking to unravel the mysteries of the human body and mind, this book offers a holistic perspective on migraines. As we embark on this exploration, may we emerge with a renewed sense of compassion, knowledge, and unity in the face of an enigmatic phenomenon that continues to shape lives in profound ways.

2. Unraveling the Science: What Causes Migraines?

Migraines are more than just severe headaches; they are complex neurological events that can significantly disrupt a person's life. For years, scientists have been delving into the intricate mechanisms behind migraines, aiming to understand the underlying causes and develop more effective treatments. While the full picture is not yet complete, researchers have made substantial progress in uncovering the science behind this enigmatic condition.

Neurovascular Interplay: The Key Player

One prominent theory in migraine research revolves around the concept of neurovascular interplay. According to this theory, migraines are initiated by changes in blood vessels and nerve pathways. The process begins with the activation of the trigeminal nerve, a major nerve responsible for sensation in the face and head. When this nerve is triggered, it releases a cascade of neurotransmitters, including serotonin and calcitonin gene-related peptide (CGRP). These substances affect the dilation and constriction of blood vessels, leading to fluctuations in blood flow to the brain.

The Role of Triggers

Triggers play a significant role in the development of migraines for many individuals. These triggers can vary widely from person to person and may include factors such as:

1. Diet: Certain foods like aged cheeses, processed meats, and foods containing additives like MSG are commonly reported triggers.

2. Environmental Factors: Bright lights, strong smells, changes in weather, and even altitude changes have been known to trigger migraines.

3. Hormonal Changes: Fluctuations in estrogen levels, such as those experienced during menstruation, pregnancy, and menopause, can influence migraine onset.

4. Stress: Emotional stress and physical tension are well-established triggers that can provoke migraine episodes.

5. Sleep Disturbances: Both inadequate sleep and oversleeping have been associated with an increased risk of migraines.

It's important to note that while triggers can provoke migraines, they are not the root cause of the condition. Rather, they act as catalysts that activate the underlying neurological processes.

Genetic Predisposition and Brain Chemistry

Genetics also appear to play a significant role in determining an individual's susceptibility to migraines. Studies have shown that if one or both parents experience migraines, their children are more likely to develop them as well. Researchers have identified several genetic variants associated with migraines, particularly those involved in regulating neurotransmitters and pain signaling.

Serotonin, a neurotransmitter with a profound impact on mood and pain perception, is of particular interest in migraine research. Imbalances in serotonin levels have been linked to the onset of migraines, and many migraine medications aim to modulate serotonin levels in the brain.

Advancements in Treatment

The multifaceted nature of migraines makes treatment a challenging endeavor. However, advances in understanding the underlying mechanisms have led to the development of more targeted therapies. Triptans, for instance, are a class of drugs that constrict blood vessels and block pain pathways. Additionally, CGRP inhibitors have shown promise in preventing migraines by targeting the key neurotransmitter involved in vasodilation and inflammation.

Lifestyle modifications, such as managing stress, maintaining a consistent sleep schedule, and identifying and avoiding personal triggers, also play a crucial role in managing migraines. These strategies, when combined with medication, can significantly improve the quality of life for individuals living with migraines.

In conclusion, the journey to unravel the science behind migraines is a dynamic and ongoing process. While much progress has been made, there is still more to learn about the intricate interplay between neurological, vascular, and genetic factors that contribute to this complex condition. As research continues, the hope is that new insights will lead to even more effective treatments and a better understanding of how to manage and ultimately prevent migraines.

3. Different Types of Migraines

Migraines are a type of headache disorder characterized by recurring episodes of severe throbbing pain, often accompanied by other symptoms such as sensitivity to light and sound, nausea, and vomiting. There are several different types of migraines, each with its own unique characteristics and triggers. Here's a comprehensive overview of the different types of migraines:

1. Migraine without Aura (Common Migraine): This is the most common type of migraine. It involves moderate to severe throbbing pain, usually on one side of the head, accompanied by symptoms such as nausea, vomiting, sensitivity to light (photophobia), and sensitivity to sound (phonophobia). It doesn't come with the warning signs known as auras.

2. Migraine with Aura (Classic Migraine): Some individuals experience auras before the onset of the headache. Auras are usually visual disturbances, such as flashing lights, zigzag lines, or blind spots. Other types of auras can involve tingling sensations in the face or extremities. The aura typically lasts for about 20 to 60 minutes and is followed by the headache phase.

3. Retinal Migraine: This rare type of migraine causes temporary vision loss or blindness in one eye. The visual symptoms can be similar to those of an aura but are limited to one eye. The vision loss is usually reversible and resolves within an hour.

4. Chronic Migraine: Chronic migraines are diagnosed when a person experiences a migraine headache on 15 or more days per month for at least three months, and at least eight of those headaches are migraines. This type can be more challenging to manage and often requires specialized treatment.

5. Menstrual Migraine: Hormonal fluctuations during the menstrual cycle can trigger migraines in some women. These

migraines occur before, during, or after menstruation and are often more severe and longer-lasting than other types of migraines.

6. Vestibular Migraine: Vestibular migraines are characterized by vertigo, dizziness, and problems with balance, in addition to the typical migraine symptoms. These episodes can be debilitating and disrupt a person's daily activities.

7. Hemiplegic Migraine: Hemiplegic migraines are rare and involve temporary paralysis or weakness on one side of the body (hemiplegia) during or after the aura phase. Other symptoms can include visual disturbances, difficulty speaking, and confusion.

8. Ophthalmic Migraine (Retinal Migraine): Often confused with retinal migraines, ophthalmic migraines cause temporary vision loss or blindness in one eye, but without the usual headache. The visual symptoms are usually accompanied by a throbbing sensation around the eye.

9. Status Migrainosus: This is a severe and prolonged migraine attack that lasts for more than 72 hours. It can be extremely debilitating and may require medical intervention to relieve the symptoms.

10. Abdominal Migraine: Primarily affecting children, abdominal migraines cause severe abdominal pain, nausea, and vomiting. These symptoms are often mistaken for gastrointestinal issues.

11. Chronic Daily Headache with Migraine Features: This type involves headaches that share characteristics with both migraines and tension-type headaches. The pain is usually moderate and can be accompanied by migraine-like symptoms.

It's important to note that accurate diagnosis and appropriate treatment are crucial for managing migraines effectively. If you suspect you are experiencing migraines or have concerns about your headaches, it's recommended to consult a healthcare professional for proper evaluation and guidance.

4. Recognizing the Symptoms: How to Diagnose Migraines

Migraines are complex and often debilitating neurological conditions that affect millions of people worldwide. Diagnosing migraines accurately is crucial for effective management and treatment. Recognizing the symptoms is the first step in this process. This article outlines the key indicators and steps to diagnose migraines.

Understanding Migraines: Migraines are more than just severe headaches. They involve a range of symptoms that can significantly impact a person's quality of life. While the exact cause of migraines is still being researched, they are believed to result from a combination of genetic and environmental factors that lead to changes in brain activity.

Common Symptoms:

1. Throbbing Headache: Migraines typically present as a pulsating or throbbing headache, often affecting one side of the head. The pain can be moderate to severe and may worsen with physical activity.

2. Sensitivity to Light and Sound: Many migraine sufferers experience heightened sensitivity to light (photophobia) and sound (phonophobia) during an attack. Normal lights and sounds may become unbearable.

3. Nausea and Vomiting: Nausea and vomiting are frequent companions of migraines. The disturbance in the digestive system is linked to the changes in brain activity during an attack.

4. Aura: Some individuals experience an aura before or during a migraine attack. Auras are usually visual disturbances like flashes of light, blind spots, or zigzag lines. However, auras can also manifest as sensory disturbances or speech difficulties.

5. Duration: Migraines can last anywhere from a few hours to several days. They tend to be more prolonged than regular headaches.

6. Triggers: Certain factors, known as triggers, can precipitate migraine attacks. Common triggers include stress, certain foods (chocolate, aged cheese, caffeine), hormonal changes, lack of sleep, and environmental factors.

Diagnosis Steps:

1. Medical History: A thorough medical history helps the healthcare provider understand your symptoms and rule out other potential causes. Be prepared to discuss the frequency, duration, and nature of your headaches.

2. Symptom Description: Accurately describing your symptoms, including the type of pain, its location, and any associated symptoms like aura, light sensitivity, and nausea, can aid in diagnosis.

3. Physical Examination: A physical examination helps the healthcare provider rule out any underlying medical conditions that might be contributing to your symptoms.

4. Diagnostic Criteria: Migraines are diagnosed based on specific criteria set by medical organizations like the International Headache Society. These criteria ensure that the symptoms meet the established guidelines for a migraine diagnosis.

5. Additional Tests: In some cases, the healthcare provider might order additional tests, such as brain imaging (MRI or CT scans), to rule out other potential causes of your symptoms.

6. Keeping a Headache Diary: Maintaining a headache diary that records the timing, duration, intensity, triggers, and any other symptoms can provide valuable insights for your healthcare provider.

Seeking Professional Help: If you suspect you have migraines or are experiencing severe headaches, it's important to seek medical attention. A healthcare professional, often a neurologist or headache specialist, can provide an accurate diagnosis and recommend an appropriate treatment plan tailored to your needs.

Conclusion: Recognizing the symptoms of migraines is crucial for an accurate diagnosis. Understanding the distinctive features of migraines and discussing them with a healthcare provider can lead to proper management and an improved quality of life for those who suffer from this condition. If you or someone you know is experiencing symptoms that align with migraines, don't hesitate to seek medical guidance.

5.Triggers and Lifestyle Factors: Identifying and Managing Precursors

In the realm of health and well-being, understanding the triggers and lifestyle factors that contribute to various conditions is crucial for early identification and effective management. By recognizing these precursors, individuals can proactively take steps to mitigate their impact and improve their overall quality of life. This article delves into the significance of identifying and managing triggers and lifestyle factors, providing insights into how they influence our health and offering strategies for prevention and intervention.

1. Triggers: Unveiling Precursors to Health Issues Triggers are stimuli or events that initiate or exacerbate health conditions. These can be internal (physiological) or external (environmental or social) factors that contribute to the development of certain health issues. Identifying triggers is essential for early intervention and preventive measures. Common triggers include:

• Environmental Factors: Pollutants, allergens, toxins, and noise pollution can trigger respiratory disorders, allergies, and stress-related conditions.

• Dietary Factors: Consuming excessive sugar, unhealthy fats, and processed foods can trigger obesity, diabetes, and cardiovascular diseases.

• Psychological Factors: Chronic stress, anxiety, and trauma can trigger mental health disorders like depression and panic disorders.

• Physical Factors: Inadequate sleep, sedentary lifestyle, and poor posture can trigger musculoskeletal issues and sleep disorders.

2. Lifestyle Factors: The Role in Precursor Management Lifestyle factors are daily habits and behaviors that significantly influence our health and well-being. By modifying these factors, individuals can manage and even prevent the development of health precursors. Key lifestyle factors include:

• Diet and Nutrition: Adopting a balanced diet rich in fruits, vegetables, whole grains, lean proteins, and healthy fats can prevent obesity, diabetes, and heart diseases.

• Physical Activity: Regular exercise reduces the risk of obesity, cardiovascular diseases, and improves mental health by promoting the release of endorphins.

• Stress Management: Engaging in relaxation techniques, meditation, and mindfulness can help mitigate the effects of chronic stress, reducing the risk of mental health issues.

• Sleep Hygiene: Prioritizing adequate and quality sleep improves cognitive function, immune response, and lowers the risk of various health conditions.

• Social Connections: Maintaining strong social ties can alleviate feelings of loneliness and depression, promoting mental well-being.

3. Identifying Precursors: Importance of Early Detection Early identification of precursors is pivotal for preventing the progression of health issues. Regular health screenings, self-assessment, and understanding family medical history can aid in recognizing potential triggers and risk factors. Timely intervention can prevent the development of chronic conditions and enable more effective treatment options.

4. Managing Precursors: Strategies for Prevention Effective management of precursors involves a holistic approach that addresses both triggers and lifestyle factors:

• Education: Raising awareness about triggers and lifestyle factors empowers individuals to make informed choices.

• Behavioral Changes: Encouraging individuals to adopt healthier habits through education and support networks can lead to sustained lifestyle improvements.

• Medical Interventions: Collaborating with healthcare professionals ensures appropriate medical interventions are implemented to manage or mitigate precursor-related risks.

• Environmental Modifications: Minimizing exposure to environmental triggers, such as pollutants or allergens, can significantly reduce health risks.

5. Long-Term Benefits: Enhanced Quality of Life Proactive management of triggers and lifestyle factors not only prevents the development of health issues but also enhances overall quality of life. By identifying and addressing precursors early on, individuals can experience

increased vitality, improved mental health, and reduced healthcare costs in the long run.

Conclusion: Recognizing triggers and lifestyle factors that contribute to health precursors is the cornerstone of preventive healthcare. By understanding these influences and taking proactive steps, individuals can effectively manage their health, prevent the onset of chronic conditions, and enjoy a higher quality of life. Empowerment through education, behavioral changes, and collaborative efforts with healthcare professionals can pave the way for a healthier and happier future.

6. Treatment Options: Medications, Therapies, and Lifestyle Changes

Migraines are severe, recurring headaches that can cause significant pain and disruption to daily life. While there is no cure for migraines, there are various treatment options available to manage and alleviate the symptoms. These options include medications, therapies, and lifestyle changes. It's important to consult a healthcare professional before starting any new treatment regimen, as they can provide personalized recommendations based on your individual needs.

1. Medications:

• Acute Pain Relief:

    • Triptans: These are a class of medications that specifically target migraine pain. They work by constricting blood vessels and blocking pain pathways in the brain.

    • Nonsteroidal Anti-Inflammatory Drugs (NSAIDs): Over-the-counter NSAIDs like ibuprofen and aspirin can provide relief by reducing inflammation and pain.

    • Acetaminophen: This pain reliever can be effective for mild to moderate migraines.

• Anti-Nausea Medications: These medications can help alleviate nausea and vomiting associated with migraines.

• Combination Medications: Some medications combine pain relievers, triptans, and anti-nausea drugs for more comprehensive relief.

• Preventive Medications:

• Beta Blockers: These medications help prevent migraines by reducing the frequency and severity of attacks.

• Antidepressants: Certain antidepressants, such as amitriptyline, can be prescribed to prevent migraines.

• Anticonvulsants: Drugs like topiramate and divalproex sodium can be effective in reducing the frequency of migraines.

2. Therapies:

• Biofeedback: This technique involves learning how to control physiological functions to manage pain and reduce migraine frequency.

• Cognitive Behavioral Therapy (CBT): CBT can help identify and manage triggers, as well as provide coping strategies for managing pain and stress.

• Physical Therapy: Therapeutic exercises and manual techniques can help relieve tension and improve posture, reducing migraine frequency.

• Acupuncture: Some individuals find relief from migraines through acupuncture, a traditional Chinese therapy involving the insertion of thin needles into specific points on the body.

• Relaxation Techniques: Techniques like deep breathing, meditation, and progressive muscle relaxation can help manage stress and reduce migraine triggers.

3. Lifestyle Changes:

• Maintain a Regular Sleep Schedule: Getting enough sleep and maintaining a consistent sleep routine can help prevent migraines.

• Stay Hydrated: Dehydration can trigger migraines in some individuals, so it's important to stay adequately hydrated.

• Dietary Changes: Identify and avoid potential trigger foods like aged cheeses, processed meats, chocolate, and artificial sweeteners.

• Stress Management: Engage in stress-reducing activities such as yoga, mindfulness, and hobbies.

• Regular Exercise: Engaging in regular physical activity can help reduce the frequency and intensity of migraines.

• Limit Caffeine and Alcohol: Both caffeine and alcohol can trigger migraines in some individuals, so moderation is key.

• Manage Hormonal Changes: For individuals whose migraines are triggered by hormonal changes, managing these fluctuations through medications or lifestyle adjustments may be helpful.

Remember that each individual's experience with migraines is unique, and the effectiveness of treatment options can vary. Consulting a healthcare professional is essential for creating a tailored treatment plan that suits your specific needs and helps you manage migraines effectively.

7.Holistic Approaches: Alternative and Complementary Therapies

Migraine, a debilitating neurological condition characterized by severe headaches, often accompanied by other symptoms like nausea, sensitivity to light and sound, can greatly impact an individual's quality of life. While conventional medical treatments can be effective, many people seek alternative and complementary therapies to manage their migraines. Holistic approaches take into account the interconnectedness of the mind, body, and environment, aiming to provide a more comprehensive and balanced approach to migraine management. Here are some alternative and complementary therapies that individuals with migraines may consider:

1. Acupuncture: This ancient Chinese practice involves inserting thin needles into specific points on the body to stimulate energy flow. Acupuncture is thought to balance the body's energy pathways and potentially alleviate migraine symptoms. Some studies suggest that regular acupuncture sessions can reduce the frequency and intensity of migraines.

2. Herbal Medicine: Certain herbs, like feverfew and butterbur, have been studied for their potential migraine-relief properties. Feverfew, in particular, is believed to reduce inflammation and relax blood vessels, possibly contributing to fewer migraine attacks. However, it's important to consult with a healthcare professional before incorporating herbal remedies into your routine.

3. Mindfulness and Meditation: Stress is a known trigger for migraines, and mindfulness techniques such as meditation, deep breathing, and progressive muscle relaxation can help manage stress and promote relaxation. Mindfulness-based stress reduction programs have shown promise in reducing the frequency and severity of migraines.

4. Yoga: Regular practice of yoga can help improve flexibility, reduce muscle tension, and alleviate stress. Some specific yoga poses and breathing exercises may be particularly beneficial for individuals with migraines by promoting relaxation and easing muscle tension.

5. Biofeedback: This technique involves using sensors to monitor physiological responses such as heart rate, skin temperature, and muscle tension. Through this real-time feedback, individuals can learn to control their body's responses, potentially reducing the frequency and intensity of migraines triggered by stress or tension.

6. Chiropractic Care: Chiropractic adjustments aim to align the spine and improve nervous system function. Some individuals with migraines report relief after chiropractic treatments, although research results are mixed. It's important to consult a qualified chiropractor and discuss your specific condition before undergoing treatment.

7. Aromatherapy: Certain essential oils, like lavender and peppermint, are believed to have calming and pain-relieving properties. Aromatherapy involves inhaling or applying these oils topically to potentially alleviate migraine symptoms. However, individual responses to

aromatherapy can vary, and caution should be exercised due to potential sensitivities.

8. Nutritional Changes: Identifying trigger foods and making dietary adjustments can play a significant role in managing migraines. Common trigger foods include caffeine, aged cheeses, processed meats, and artificial sweeteners. Maintaining a balanced and nutritious diet, staying hydrated, and avoiding potential triggers can contribute to migraine prevention.

9. Physical Therapy: Muscular imbalances and poor posture can contribute to migraines. A physical therapist can assess your posture, muscle tension, and movement patterns, and develop a customized exercise and stretching plan to address these issues.

10. Tai Chi: This mind-body practice involves slow, flowing movements and deep breathing. It has been associated with reduced stress, improved balance, and overall well-being. Engaging in regular Tai Chi practice may help manage migraine triggers related to stress and tension.

It's essential to remember that individual responses to these holistic approaches can vary widely. Before beginning any new therapy or treatment, especially if you have an existing medical condition or are taking medication, it's crucial to consult with a qualified healthcare professional. Integrating holistic therapies into a comprehensive migraine management plan, in collaboration with medical advice, can help individuals find a balanced and effective approach to reducing the impact of migraines on their lives.

8.Coping Strategies: Navigating Migraines in Daily Life

Coping with migraines can be challenging, but having effective strategies in place can help you navigate daily life more comfortably. Here are some coping strategies to consider:

1. Identify Triggers: Keep a detailed migraine diary to track potential triggers such as foods, beverages, stressors, sleep patterns, weather changes, and hormonal fluctuations. Identifying triggers can help you avoid or manage them better.

2. Maintain a Routine: Stick to a consistent daily routine for sleep, meals, and physical activity. Erratic schedules can trigger migraines, so maintaining stability can be beneficial.

3. Stay Hydrated: Dehydration can be a migraine trigger for some people. Drink plenty of water throughout the day to keep your body well-hydrated.

4. Prioritize Sleep: Aim for a consistent sleep schedule and create a comfortable sleep environment. Poor sleep can exacerbate migraines, so getting enough quality rest is crucial.

5. Practice Stress Management: Stress is a common migraine trigger. Engage in relaxation techniques such as deep breathing, meditation, yoga, or mindfulness to help manage stress levels.

6. Dietary Modifications: Some individuals find relief by making dietary changes. Avoiding potential trigger foods

like caffeine, chocolate, aged cheeses, and processed meats could help reduce migraine occurrences.

7. Medication and Supplements: Work with your healthcare provider to develop a medication plan. Over-the-counter pain relievers or prescription medications specifically designed for migraines might be beneficial. Some people also find relief with magnesium supplements or riboflavin (vitamin B2).

8. Caffeine Management: While caffeine can provide relief for some during a migraine, it can trigger migraines in others. Moderation and consistency in your caffeine intake might help.

9. Regular Exercise: Engage in regular, moderate exercise, as it can help reduce the frequency and severity of migraines. Avoid intense workouts during peak migraine periods.

10. Stay Prepared: Carry a small bag with essentials like medication, sunglasses, a hat, and a water bottle. Being prepared can help you manage unexpected migraines when you're away from home.

11. Stay in a Dark, Quiet Environment: When a migraine strikes, find a calm, dark, and quiet space to rest until it passes. This can help alleviate discomfort and sensitivity to light and noise.

12. Use Cold Compresses: Applying a cold or cool compress to your forehead or the back of your neck can provide relief by constricting blood vessels and reducing inflammation.

13. Mindfulness and Relaxation: Engage in deep breathing exercises, progressive muscle relaxation, or guided imagery to redirect your focus away from the pain and help your body relax.

14. Social Support: Communicate with family, friends, and colleagues about your condition. Their understanding and support can make it easier to manage migraines in social situations.

15. Professional Help: If your migraines significantly impact your daily life, consider working with a neurologist, pain specialist, or headache clinic to develop a comprehensive treatment plan.

Remember that everyone's experience with migraines is unique, so it may take time to discover which coping strategies work best for you. Consistency and patience are key as you navigate life with migraines.

9.Migraines and Mental Health: Understanding the Connection

Migraines are more than just intense headaches. They are a complex neurological condition that affects millions of people worldwide, often causing debilitating pain, sensory disturbances, and various other symptoms. However, what many people might not realize is that migraines and mental health are intricately connected. This article delves into the relationship between migraines and mental health, exploring how one can impact the other and offering insights into managing both aspects for a better quality of life.

The Bidirectional Relationship

1. Impact of Migraines on Mental Health: Migraines can significantly affect mental health due to the nature of the condition. The chronic pain, frequent attacks, and unpredictable nature of migraines can lead to a range of emotional and psychological challenges:

• Anxiety and Panic: The fear of when the next migraine attack will occur can trigger anxiety and panic attacks in individuals who suffer from migraines. The uncertainty surrounding their daily lives can lead to heightened stress levels.

• Depression: Chronic pain and the disruption of daily activities due to migraines can contribute to feelings of helplessness, isolation, and sadness. This emotional toll can lead to or exacerbate depression in some individuals.

• Reduced Quality of Life: Migraines can restrict social interactions, limit participation in activities, and affect work or school performance. These limitations can negatively impact self-esteem and overall life satisfaction.

2. Impact of Mental Health on Migraines: Mental health conditions can also influence the frequency and severity of migraine attacks:

• Stress as a Trigger: Stress is a common trigger for migraines. High stress levels can lead to physiological changes that increase the likelihood of migraine attacks. This creates a feedback loop where stress triggers migraines, and migraines, in turn, lead to more stress.

• Anxiety and Tension: Mental health issues such as generalized anxiety disorder can cause muscle tension and contribute to the development of tension-type headaches, which are often mistaken for migraines.

• Coping Mechanisms: Individuals with mental health challenges might resort to unhealthy coping mechanisms, such as overusing painkillers or caffeine, which can worsen migraines over time.

Managing the Connection

1. Holistic Approaches: Treating migraines and addressing mental health should be holistic. Integrating the following strategies can improve both aspects of well-being:

• Stress Management: Practicing relaxation techniques, mindfulness, meditation, and regular exercise can help mitigate the impact of stress on migraines and mental health.

• Healthy Lifestyle: Prioritizing a balanced diet, regular sleep patterns, and staying hydrated can contribute to reducing the frequency and severity of migraine attacks.

• Therapy: Cognitive-behavioral therapy (CBT) and other forms of psychotherapy can help individuals develop coping strategies to manage the emotional impact of migraines.

• Medication and Consultation: Consultation with healthcare professionals is essential. They can provide medications to manage migraines and refer individuals to mental health specialists if needed.

2. Building Support Systems: Building a strong support system can be crucial for managing both migraines and mental health challenges:

• Communication: Openly discussing the challenges with friends, family, and employers can lead to a better understanding of the condition and garner necessary support.

• Support Groups: Participating in support groups or online communities can help individuals connect with others who are experiencing similar challenges, reducing feelings of isolation.

The connection between migraines and mental health is a complex interplay that requires a comprehensive approach to management. By recognizing the bidirectional relationship between these two aspects, individuals can take steps to manage both their migraines and mental health more effectively, leading to a better overall quality of life. It is important to consult healthcare professionals for tailored guidance and support in addressing these challenges.

10. Migraines in Specific Groups: Children, Adolescents, Women, and Seniors

Migraines can affect various demographic groups differently, leading to distinct challenges and considerations. Here's an overview of how migraines manifest in specific groups: children, adolescents, women, and seniors.

1. Children: Migraines in children are often underdiagnosed due to difficulties in communication. Common symptoms include intense head pain, nausea, vomiting, and sensitivity to light and sound. Children may have difficulty describing their symptoms accurately, making it essential for parents and caregivers to be vigilant. Migraines can disrupt school attendance, social interactions, and overall quality of life. Identifying triggers, managing stress, and maintaining a regular routine can help mitigate migraines in children.

2. Adolescents: Adolescents experiencing migraines might face challenges in their academic and social lives. Hormonal fluctuations, stress, irregular sleep patterns, and dietary habits can trigger migraines. Proper diagnosis is crucial, as migraines can be mistaken for tension headaches or other issues. Education about triggers and lifestyle modifications, along with stress management techniques, can empower adolescents to manage their migraines effectively.

3. Women: Hormonal fluctuations, particularly during menstruation, pregnancy, and menopause, make women more susceptible to migraines. Menstrual migraines often

occur just before or during a woman's period. Pregnancy can bring relief for some women, while exacerbating symptoms for others. Medication options need to be carefully considered, especially during pregnancy. Women with migraines should work closely with their healthcare providers to create a comprehensive management plan that addresses hormonal triggers.

4. Seniors: Migraines can persist into old age or develop anew in seniors. Differentiating migraines from other age-related health issues can be challenging. Seniors may also experience cognitive impairment, complicating accurate diagnosis. Treatment plans should consider existing medical conditions and potential interactions with other medications. Seniors might face additional challenges due to limited mobility, making self-care and symptom management more complex. Lifestyle adjustments, preventive measures, and appropriate pain management strategies are vital in this age group.

In conclusion, migraines can manifest differently in various demographic groups, necessitating tailored approaches to diagnosis, management, and treatment. Understanding the unique challenges and triggers specific to each group can lead to better outcomes and improved quality of life for individuals affected by migraines. If you or someone you know experiences migraines, seeking medical advice and creating a personalized plan is essential.

11. Work and Migraines: Strategies for Managing Professional Life

Migraines are debilitating and disruptive headaches that can have a significant impact on one's personal and professional life. For individuals who experience migraines, managing their symptoms while maintaining a successful career can be challenging. This guide aims to provide practical strategies for effectively navigating the intersection of work and migraines, enabling individuals to achieve their professional goals while prioritizing their health and well-being.

1. Understanding Migraines: It's crucial to comprehend the nature of migraines, their triggers, and the different stages they go through. This understanding will help in identifying warning signs and planning accordingly.

2. Open Communication: Inform your employer, supervisor, and colleagues about your migraines. Transparency can lead to increased empathy and support. Discuss potential accommodations, such as flexible work hours or a quiet workspace, to minimize triggers and manage symptoms.

3. Time Management: Efficiently manage your time by breaking down tasks into manageable chunks. Prioritize tasks and create a realistic schedule, allowing for regular breaks to prevent stress-induced migraines.

4. Work Environment: Tailor your workspace to your needs. Ensure proper lighting, minimize noise, and

maintain ergonomic arrangements to prevent migraines triggered by sensory factors.

5. Stress Management: Stress is a common migraine trigger. Practice stress-reduction techniques such as deep breathing, meditation, yoga, and regular exercise to mitigate its effects.

6. Hydration and Nutrition: Stay well-hydrated and maintain a balanced diet. Avoid trigger foods, such as caffeine, alcohol, and processed foods, that could exacerbate migraines.

7. Sleep Routine: Establish a consistent sleep routine, aiming for 7-9 hours of quality sleep each night. Adequate rest can significantly reduce the frequency and severity of migraines.

8. Medication and Treatment Plan: Consult a healthcare professional to develop a comprehensive treatment plan. This may include prescribed medications, preventive measures, and strategies for managing acute attacks.

9. Flexible Work Arrangements: Explore options like remote work or flexible hours to accommodate your migraine patterns. Having the ability to adapt your work environment can enhance your productivity and reduce triggers.

10. Utilize Technology: Leverage technology to your advantage. Use task management apps, noise-canceling headphones, blue light filters, and ergonomic tools to minimize strain on your senses.

11. Emergency Plan: Have an emergency plan in place for severe migraine episodes. Communicate this plan to your supervisor and colleagues so they understand the steps to take in case of an emergency.

12. Self-Care: Prioritize self-care to manage migraines better. Engage in activities that bring you joy, relax your mind, and promote overall well-being.

Conclusion: Balancing a professional career with migraines requires careful planning, open communication, and a proactive approach to health. By implementing these strategies, individuals can effectively manage their migraines while still pursuing their career goals. Remember that your health comes first, and finding the right balance between work and well-being is key to long-term success and happiness.

12. Relationships and Support: Communicating about Migraines with Loved Ones

Migraines are more than just headaches; they are complex neurological conditions that can significantly impact a person's life. When dealing with migraines, open and effective communication with loved ones becomes crucial. Sharing your experiences, needs, and feelings can foster understanding and support, helping you navigate through challenging times together. This article provides insights into communicating about migraines with your loved ones, fostering a supportive environment that promotes empathy and cooperation.

1. Educate Your Loved Ones: Begin by educating your loved ones about migraines. Explain that migraines are not just regular headaches, but rather a multifaceted condition involving sensory sensitivities, visual disturbances, and often debilitating pain. Providing them with accurate information can dispel misconceptions and help them understand the severity of your situation.

2. Express Your Experience: Describe your migraine experience to your loved ones in detail. Share the symptoms you typically experience, such as aura, intense pain, nausea, and sensitivity to light and sound. Let them know how migraines impact your daily activities, productivity, and overall quality of life.

3. Share Triggers and Warning Signs: Inform your loved ones about the triggers that can lead to migraines. These triggers could include certain foods, stress, hormonal changes, lack of sleep, or environmental factors. Explain the warning signs you notice before a migraine attack, so they can recognize when you might need extra support or accommodations.

4. Communicate Needs and Limitations: Clearly communicate your needs and limitations during migraine episodes. Let your loved ones know if you need a quiet and dark space, rest, or specific medications. Discuss potential adjustments they can make to create a more comfortable environment for you during these times.

5. Develop a Plan Together: Collaborate with your loved ones to create a plan for dealing with migraines. Discuss how you would like them to respond when you're experiencing an attack. Establish a system for communicating your needs, whether it's through a specific phrase or signal, so they can offer assistance without causing additional stress.

6. Acknowledge Emotional Impact: Migraines can take an emotional toll, leading to frustration, anxiety, and even depression. Let your loved ones know how these emotional aspects affect you. Encourage open conversations about your feelings and reassure them that your mood changes are a part of the migraine experience.

7. Practice Empathy and Patience: Encourage your loved ones to practice empathy and patience. Migraines can be unpredictable, and recovery times may vary. Help them

understand that your condition is not something you can control entirely, and setbacks can happen.

8. Offer Resources: Share reliable resources about migraines with your loved ones. This could include articles, videos, or support groups where they can learn more about the condition and gain insights from others who are dealing with similar situations.

9. Celebrate Small Victories: Celebrate together when you have good days or successfully manage a migraine episode. This can create a positive atmosphere and help both you and your loved ones focus on progress and resilience.

10. Reevaluate and Adjust: Regularly reevaluate your communication and support strategies. Ask your loved ones for feedback and be open to adjusting your approach based on their insights. This ongoing dialogue can strengthen your relationship and enhance the effectiveness of your support network.

Communicating about migraines with loved ones is essential for fostering understanding, empathy, and support. By sharing your experiences, educating them about the condition, and working together to create a plan, you can build a strong foundation that helps you navigate the challenges of living with migraines as a united front. Remember, open communication is key to developing a network of care that can make a significant difference in your journey.

13. Future Directions: Emerging Research and Innovations

Migraine is a complex neurological disorder characterized by recurring moderate to severe headaches, often accompanied by symptoms such as nausea, sensitivity to light and sound, and in some cases, visual disturbances known as auras. While significant progress has been made in understanding migraine triggers, mechanisms, and treatment options, there is still much to explore and discover. This article delves into the potential future directions of migraine research and the innovations that might shape the landscape of migraine management.

1. Genomics and Personalized Medicine: Advancements in genomic research have the potential to uncover specific genetic markers associated with migraine susceptibility and severity. As we gain a deeper understanding of the genetic basis of migraines, personalized treatment plans tailored to an individual's genetic profile could become a reality. This could lead to more effective preventative strategies and targeted therapies.

2. Neuroimaging and Brain Connectivity: Functional MRI (fMRI) and other advanced neuroimaging techniques can

provide insights into the altered brain connectivity patterns during migraine attacks. Future research might focus on using these techniques to identify specific brain regions and networks involved in different phases of migraines, helping us understand the underlying mechanisms and potentially guiding novel treatments.

3. Neuroinflammation and Immune System Involvement: There's growing evidence of neuroinflammatory processes contributing to migraine pathophysiology. Exploring the relationship between the immune system and migraine attacks could pave the way for new anti-inflammatory treatments. Targeting specific immune pathways might offer novel strategies for preventing and treating migraines.

4. Digital Health and Wearable Technologies: Wearable devices capable of monitoring physiological parameters, such as heart rate variability, skin temperature, and brain activity, could provide real-time insights into an individual's migraine patterns. Analyzing this data might help predict and manage impending migraine attacks, empowering patients to take timely preventive measures.

5. Neuromodulation Techniques: Non-invasive neuromodulation methods, such as transcranial magnetic stimulation (TMS) and transcutaneous electrical nerve stimulation (TENS), are being explored as potential migraine treatments. As our understanding of the brain's electrical and magnetic fields grows, these techniques could offer non-pharmacological alternatives for both acute and preventive migraine management.

6. Gut-Brain Axis and Microbiome Research: The gut-brain axis has gained attention for its potential role in various neurological disorders, including migraines. Emerging research suggests that the gut microbiome might influence migraine occurrence through the modulation of systemic inflammation and neurotransmitter production. Investigating this link could reveal new therapeutic avenues.

7. Neuroplasticity and Behavioral Interventions: Understanding the brain's ability to rewire itself (neuroplasticity) opens doors for behavioral interventions. Cognitive-behavioral therapy, mindfulness, and biofeedback techniques could help migraine sufferers manage pain perception, stress, and triggers, ultimately reducing the frequency and intensity of attacks.

8. Drug Development and Targeted Therapies: Continued research into migraine-specific drug targets and mechanisms could lead to the development of more effective and better-tolerated medications. New classes of drugs, such as CGRP (calcitonin gene-related peptide) inhibitors, have already shown promise. Future innovations might involve combining these agents with other treatments for enhanced efficacy.

 The landscape of migraine research and treatment is rapidly evolving, driven by breakthroughs in genetics, neuroscience, digital health, and innovative therapeutic approaches. As our understanding of migraine mechanisms deepens, the potential for more personalized, effective, and holistic management strategies holds great promise for improving the quality of life for millions of migraine sufferers worldwide.

14. Building a Migraine Management Plan: A Step-by-Step Guide

Living with migraines can be challenging, but with a well-structured management plan, you can take control of your symptoms and improve your quality of life. This step-by-step guide will help you build an effective migraine management plan tailored to your needs.

Step 1: Educate Yourself About Migraines Understanding the nature of migraines is crucial for effective management. Research the causes, triggers, symptoms, and different types of migraines. Knowledge empowers you to make informed decisions about your health.

Step 2: Consult a Healthcare Professional Seek guidance from a healthcare provider, preferably a neurologist or headache specialist, who can accurately diagnose your condition and provide personalized recommendations. Discuss your medical history, symptoms, and any treatments you've tried before.

Step 3: Identify Triggers Keep a detailed migraine diary to track your attacks and potential triggers such as foods, stress, hormonal changes, weather, and sleep patterns. Identifying triggers can help you avoid or minimize them in the future.

Step 4: Develop a Treatment Plan Based on your healthcare provider's recommendations, create a comprehensive treatment plan that may include:

• Acute Medications: Over-the-counter or prescription medications for managing pain and associated symptoms during an attack.

• Preventive Medications: Prescription drugs taken daily to reduce the frequency and intensity of migraines.

• Lifestyle Modifications: Implement changes in your routine, diet, sleep patterns, and stress management techniques to reduce the occurrence of migraines.

• Alternative Therapies: Consider complementary approaches such as acupuncture, biofeedback, or relaxation techniques.

Step 5: Establish a Routine Consistency is key to managing migraines. Stick to a regular sleep schedule, meal times, and stress-reduction practices. Maintain hydration and avoid skipping meals.

Step 6: Incorporate Stress Management Stress is a common migraine trigger. Practice stress reduction techniques such as deep breathing, meditation, yoga, or progressive muscle relaxation.

Step 7: Maintain a Healthy Diet Certain foods can trigger migraines in susceptible individuals. Keep a balanced diet, avoiding known trigger foods like aged cheeses, processed meats, and artificial sweeteners.

Step 8: Stay Hydrated Dehydration can trigger migraines. Drink enough water throughout the day and limit caffeine and alcohol intake.

Step 9: Regular Exercise Engage in regular, moderate exercise to improve overall health and reduce the frequency of migraines. Avoid intense workouts during migraine attacks.

Step 10: Monitor and Adjust Regularly assess the effectiveness of your management plan. Note any changes in migraine frequency, intensity, or triggers. Discuss your progress with your healthcare provider and make necessary adjustments to your plan.

Creating a personalized migraine management plan takes dedication and patience. By understanding your triggers, adopting a healthy lifestyle, and working closely with your healthcare provider, you can take significant steps toward minimizing the impact of migraines on your life. Remember that each person's experience is unique, so your management plan should be tailored to your specific needs and preferences.

15. Advocacy and Awareness: Joining the Migraine Community

Migraines are more than just headaches; they are complex neurological disorders that can significantly impact a person's quality of life. Whether you're someone who suffers from migraines or simply wishes to support those who do, joining the migraine community can make a difference. Advocacy and awareness play crucial roles in improving understanding, research, and treatment options for those affected by migraines. In this article, we will explore the importance of joining the migraine community, how to get involved, and the positive impact you can have.

Understanding Migraines:

Migraines are characterized by intense throbbing pain, often on one side of the head, and can be accompanied by symptoms like nausea, sensitivity to light and sound, and even visual disturbances. They affect millions of people worldwide, causing missed workdays, disrupted routines, and a general decrease in overall well-being. By joining the migraine community, you become a part of the effort to raise awareness about the complexities of this condition and advocate for better support systems.

Why Join the Migraine Community:

1. Support Network: Connecting with others who understand your struggles can provide invaluable emotional support. Whether you're a migraine sufferer or a supporter, sharing experiences, tips, and coping strategies can foster a sense of belonging and lessen the isolation often felt by those with migraines.

2. Advocacy: The migraine community is a powerful force for advocacy. By joining, you add your voice to the call for increased research funding, improved treatment options, and better workplace accommodations for migraine sufferers. Together, we can influence policies and practices that affect the lives of millions.

3. Awareness: Migraine awareness is essential for dispelling myths and misconceptions surrounding the condition. Joining the community allows you to educate others about what migraines really are, how they impact lives, and how everyone can contribute to a more inclusive and understanding society.

Getting Involved:

1. Online Communities: There are numerous online forums, social media groups, and websites dedicated to migraines. These platforms allow you to connect with fellow sufferers, share experiences, and stay updated on the latest research and treatment options.

2. Local Support Groups: Check if there are local support groups or meet-ups in your area. Meeting face-to-face

with others who understand can provide a unique sense of camaraderie and shared purpose.

3. Advocacy Organizations: Many organizations, such as the Migraine Research Foundation and the American Migraine Foundation, actively work to raise awareness and promote research. Consider volunteering, donating, or participating in their advocacy campaigns.

4. Educational Initiatives: Host or participate in events that aim to educate your community about migraines. This could include informational sessions at local schools, workplaces, or community centers.

Making an Impact:

1. Spread Awareness: Share accurate information about migraines on your social media platforms, using relevant hashtags to increase visibility. This helps combat misconceptions and provides valuable resources for those seeking help.

2. Advocate for Change: Write to your local representatives, urging them to support legislation that aids migraine sufferers, such as better healthcare coverage and workplace accommodations.

3. Participate in Fundraising: Support research efforts by participating in fundraising events, walks, or runs organized by advocacy organizations.

4. Share Personal Stories: Personal stories have the power to humanize the experience of migraines. Consider sharing your own story to inspire others and foster empathy within the community.

Joining the migraine community is not just about supporting those who suffer from this condition; it's about creating a more inclusive, informed, and compassionate society. By advocating for better treatment options, spreading awareness, and offering support, you contribute to a collective effort that can transform the lives of millions. Whether you're a migraine sufferer or an empathetic ally, your involvement matters. Together, we can make strides towards a future with better understanding and improved quality of life for those affected by migraines.

16. Resources and References: Where to Find Reliable Information

Certainly, here are some reliable resources and references where you can find information about migraines:

1. American Migraine Foundation (AMF): Website: https://americanmigrainefoundation.org/ The AMF provides comprehensive information about migraines, including causes, symptoms, triggers, treatment options, and lifestyle management.

2. Migraine Trust: Website: https://www.migrainetrust.org/ This UK-based organization offers valuable resources, research updates, and support for individuals affected by migraines.

3. Mayo Clinic: Website: https://www.mayoclinic.org/diseases-conditions/migraine-headache/ Mayo Clinic provides authoritative information on various health conditions, including migraine causes, symptoms, diagnosis, and treatment options.

4. National Institute of Neurological Disorders and Stroke (NINDS): Website: https://www.ninds.nih.gov/Disorders/All-Disorders/Migraine-Information-Page NINDS offers information on migraine research, clinical trials, and treatment approaches.

5. WebMD: Website: https://www.webmd.com/migraines-headaches/default.htm WebMD provides easy-to-understand information about migraines, their causes, triggers, treatments, and prevention strategies.

6. Migraine.com: Website: https://migraine.com/ Migraine.com offers a platform for individuals to share their experiences, find community support, and access information about migraines.

7. PubMed: Website: https://pubmed.ncbi.nlm.nih.gov/ A comprehensive database of biomedical literature, PubMed provides access to research articles, studies, and clinical trials related to migraines and headache disorders.

8. Cochrane Library: Website: https://www.cochranelibrary.com/ The Cochrane Library offers systematic reviews and evidence-based information on healthcare topics, including migraine treatments.

9. Neurology Journals: Journals like Cephalalgia, Headache, and Neurology often publish research articles, studies, and clinical insights related to migraines and headache disorders.

10. Local and National Health Organizations: Organizations such as the World Health Organization (WHO), Centers for